Dr. Cargill's Natural European Facelift and Rejuvenation

Dr. Cargill

Published by Acie Cargill
aciecargill@gmail.com
http://aciecargill.com

ISBN-13:978-1721635535
ISBN-10:172163553X

Formatted - Brenda Van Niekerk
brenda@triomarketers.com

Website Design - Brenda Van Niekerk
http://triomarketers.com

Synopsis

Dr. Cargill learned the technique of European natural face rejuvenation from 3 distinguished physicians from the last generation, Dr. Paavo Airola, Dr. Rose Arvigo, and Dr. Loretta Hilschur. After many years of doing the facial work on patients, Dr. Cargill decided to write down the techniques and materials that he uses and make the information available to the next generation.

The facial work can be done on yourself. It is not quite as effective as having a skilled practitioner do it, but it will work doing it on yourself. Be careful on the preparations of the herbs and oils and follow the directions exactly. Pay particular attention to the work on the face muscles and the cleansing of the skin.

Ageing is normal, to an extent, but if your appearance can be remarkably improved by following the directions in this little book, then why not do it? Throw away your makeup and let your face and neck glow with natural health and stronger face muscles lifted into a more youthful position. When you look better, you will feel better.

Table of Contents

1. Introduction

Some years ago, when I was a young man, I went to Germany and studied at a seminar on facial work with Dr. Paavo Airola, the greatest naturopath of his time. I also studied with naprapaths and herbalists Dr. Rosita Arvigo and Dr. Loretta Hilschur, both noted in their fields.

I did the facials myself for many years and I was always amazed at the results. Even on men. In fact, most of my facial patients were men, but their faces are often coarse and have scar tissue and are more difficult to work with, but this treatment does help them also.

You can give yourself the facial treatment. It is not quite as effective as having a skilled practitioner do it for you. There is something healing about the touch of another person's hands, but if that is not available to you, then do it to yourself. Make your face look younger and fresher and you will feel better because you look better.

Ageing changes us. It seems like our minds stay younger longer, but our appearance naturally deteriorates with age. Our face muscles sag because we don't use them in beneficial ways. Many of the facial muscles are embedded in the skin of the face.

As they get weak, we look older. You can cover it up with makeup or you can just accept looking older or you can give yourself a series of the natural facelifts and rejuvenation.

It takes a little time. You must do the muscle stretching and strengthening and you have to prepare the herbal pack. You have to find a source for the fresh herbs. I grow my own. They are easy to grow. And you should do a treatment twice a week for several months. You will look ten years younger. At least.

Follow the directions exactly. Everything is natural. Absolutely no harmful chemicals or synthetics. Natural herbs and oils.

And you will need to find your own clay for an occasional mask. Make sure the clay is all natural. We are making your skin extremely clean and receptive and I don't want you putting any kind of chemical on your face. So read the ingredients on the clay carefully and choose the one with the least ingredients. I prefer 100% all-natural clay especially prepared for facial work.

The oils are very important. I prefer Dr. Airola's own mixture which is listed in the book. You will need to find 100% pure cold-pressed sesame oil either at a health food store or a seller on the internet. And organic kelp granules and organic oat flakes. Then you are ready to get started on your way to a restoration of your original beauty. Go for it. Be beautiful. Why not!!!

2. Clay mask

This is an optional part of the therapy. It does not need to be done every time you do the facial treatment. Maybe once every two weeks or even just once a month. It does draw out a lot of impurities blocking the pores of the skin and if you use a pure clay, it will not harm your skin, but you do not have to use it very often.

Get pure clay. No additives or chemicals on your face. The mildest clay for sensitive, dry skin is white Kaolin clay, the French Green clay is for oily skin, and Moroccan Rhassoul clay is probably the strongest and draws the best. Mix about a tablespoon in a container with some pure water and make a fairly thick mixture. One of the best ways to apply it is with a small cooking brush. Let it dry for no more than 20 minutes, maybe only 8 to 10 minutes your first time. Maybe a little less if it is uncomfortable. Some therapists use a slice of cucumber over each eye and it seems like a good idea. Then scrape the clay off and wash your skin thoroughly with pure water and a sponge

3. The Massage

First clean the face with pure water. Not tap water. We want no chlorine on your face and no soap. Just pure water on a sponge and clean it good. Now put a small amount of cold-pressed sesame oil on your palms and fronts of your fingers.

Move your hands across your forehead and down the sides of your face and do your neck also and under your chin. Put your hands on either side of your nose and slide your hands to the sides. Stroke all around your eyes and the eyelids. Repeat these movements at least five times.

Bend your two index fingers and do light pinching movements between the index fingers and pad of your thumbs. All over your face and neck at least five times. Now do the pinching with a twist of the skin several times all over your face.

Use the pads of your open fingers to lightly and rapidly tap your face all over for a few minutes.

Now use your open hands to stroke your neck and face going upwards. Again and again. All over your face. Let's get an exchange of blood. Get the old blood out and new blood in. Your blood will heal your face. Make you young again. The more massage of your face and neck, the better. It is a wonderful therapy. Heal yourself with your own hands. Or teach someone else to do it for you. Now take a towel and wipe your face clean from the oil.

4. Face muscle work

Weak muscles cause the face to sag and look older. Let's try to stretch the muscles and make them stronger and healthier so that the face pulls back into its normal position. I will just cover 6 main stretches, but if your client or friend or yourself has a particular facial problem you can use the same principles on that facial muscle also.

The main work is to stretch the muscle and then resist pulling it back. That is how the muscles are strengthened and after several sessions they will begin to assume a more natural and younger appearance. Sagging muscles will be strengthened and many wrinkles can be helped before they become more difficult with scar tissue in them.

First of all, go over the entire face with clean warm water on a sponge. Then do nice drainage strokes with your open hand followed by little pinches and twists to break up scar tissue beginning to form and get some blood in the skin and superficial muscles.

The strengthening principles are the same for all facial muscle groups and actually is the same for every muscle in the body. Stretch and resist. The stretching might make you feel the face is going in the wrong direction, but like for any muscle, this is how you strengthen them. Stretch the muscle to its fullest extent and then resist when you are bringing it back. Just resist enough to exercise the muscle.

The muscle will naturally move back to its original position, but now it will be strengthened and will lift against the force of gravity that was causing your face to sag. A stretched muscle is a stronger muscle and will eventually lead to a younger and healthier appearance. Stretch then resist. Here are 6 main muscle groups that probably need attention.

1. <u>Frontalis.</u> This is the muscle under the skin of the forehead. Press down at the eyebrows and stretch. Now lift the eyebrows upwards while you resist. Keep resisting all the way up and them do it again. Stretch and then resist. Try it at least 10 times. You are exercising the muscles that move the forehead. Move the fingers to different spots on the eyebrows when you stretch. Then some nice strokes up and down and across the forehead with the open hand. Work the forehead with your fingers going in circles. Bring new blood to that muscle and nourish it. Make it healthy. And it will make you beautiful.

2. <u>Oris.</u> These muscles go around the mouth to pucker the lips. Stretch the pucker to maximum between your thumb and fingers and then resist

bringing it back. Do it at least 5 times then some nice strokes in all directions around the mouth.

3. <u>Risorius</u> these muscles pull the corners of the mouth open for a big smile. Stretch the smile with the thumb and middle finger and resist bringing it back. At least, 5 times and then cleansing strokes to bring in fresh blood for the muscles.

4. <u>Masticators</u> are on the side of your cheeks near the jaw line, so stretch the mouth wide open with your thumb and index finger on your chin and resist bringing the jaw back up. Then stretch again a little further open. Then resist closing again. These muscles are very important for your appearance. Maybe do this stretch 10 times.

5. <u>Buccinators</u> are on the sides of the cheeks closer to the nose. They assist in chewing food and are very important to a youthful appearance. Blow up your cheeks as much as you can then place one finger on each of your cheeks with your mouth closed. Then resist trying to blow the air out of your cheeks. Do this at least 10 times and each time try to blow up your cheeks a little more.

6. <u>Neck Muscles</u> there are many muscles in the neck, but I am just concerned here with those in front from about the corners of jaw down to your collar bones. These muscles get weak and cause your neck to be

flabby looking. Here is how to strengthen them for a more youthful appearance. Put the back of your fingers underneath your jaw and stretch the whole jaw upwards, then resist bringing the jaw down. Now stretch the jaw upward again and this time go a little further up. Now resist lowering the jaw again. Repeat ten times. Now drainage strokes on your neck with the flat part of your hand moving the blood towards your heart.

What do I think of a TENS unit to stimulate the facial muscles? They are reasonably priced $25-$50 (and can also be used for pain relief). A TENS unit cannot stimulate the larger deeper muscles, but for the muscles that are near the surface of the skin of the face and neck, I think the TENS unit will strengthen them. Try it. Learn the settings and the correct pad placements and you will get an electronic facelift.

5. The Cleansing

Your facial skin is caked with bacteria, dead skin, oils, and a variety of dirt and impurities. Sorry. That's just the way it is. Everything is caked on microscopically. It is surprising the amount of microorganisms like bacteria and fungi fighting for a spot. Your skin is covered almost completely. And that doesn't matter how much you wash your face or what type of cleansers. It is normal flora and over the millions of years we have been on earth, we have adapted to being covered with microorganisms.

So how are we going to work on your skin if it is covered with bacteria and other almost invisible living things. Well, first of all, the barrier they present is not completely impregnable. They are close together but not touching totally. Otherwise, our skin could not really live and function as skin. Plus, we are going to treat the face with a mild herbal antibiotic that hopefully will thin them out somewhat. I don't like using anything unnatural on your face. So I don't want to use the synthetic antibiotics sold in drug stores.

There are several herbs with good antibiotic properties. My two favorites are golden seal and echinacea. Get a small package of the root of the plant and make a decoction. Actually boil a teaspoon of the root in a glass or ceramic pot for 15 minutes. After it cools, use a cotton ball and apply it all over the face. Do this for at least five minutes and you have to be sort of vigorous to dislodge the bacteria. When you are done, throw away the liquid you were dipping into, but refrigerate your main herbal decoction in an airtight container for future use.

Now, let's wash your face with clear water and a sponge. Do not use soap the day of a facial. Just clear water. Rinse out the sponge often and go over your face again and again. You may have to change the water, even if it looks clean. You should be wearing a shower cap and keep your hair pulled back so you can wash right up to your hairline. Take your time, this is a very important step and it will help relax all those face muscles in your skin.

Soak some organic oat flakes in a dish with water and dab the liquid all over your face with a cotton ball. Then cut a piece of an old nylon panty hose and fold it over with organic kelp granules in it. Dip it in the water and scrub your face. Clean out those clogged pores and blemishes. Save the nylon with the kelp. We will use it again.

Use cold-pressed sesame oil on a cotton ball and clean the whole face. Everywhere, especially on your nose and neck. Cleanse with fresh water again with the sponge. Now use a small wet loofa to scrape off dead cells and debris and some bacteria also. Do it firmly. Take your time. This is important. Then rinse with cold water again with a sponge. Redo the oatmeal water and the kelp scrub and the sesame oil. One more rinsing with the water and sponge. You are ready for the herbal pack.

6. The Herbal Pack

You can use most any cloth, but preferably, natural white pure cotton. That is what I would use if I am just doing one facial, like if I was just doing myself, but if you are doing multiple facials, it is a lot of cloths and cleaning. I had good results using throw away diapers like pampers and just cut a small breathing hole for the nostrils. When you are done recycle it.

I have a special chair designed so the patient can be sitting and the back lowers into a reclining position with the head supported and the face pointing up. I think it is advantageous for the patient to be sort of laying back like in a supine position because it is comfortable, and the patient will be in that position for 30 to 40 minutes. Sitting up can work, but it is not preferable because the herbal liquid will probably drain away from the face.

A bed or a couch can also work but you will have to find a way to protect the furniture from the liquid which will probably spill out from the pack. Or use the floor if it can be made comfortable. Something like a massage table would be ideal because the patient will be available at the right height. I know someone who uses three armless kitchen chairs in a row and that makes a functional work table for the patient to lie upon.

It is necessary to extract the active principles from the herbs we are going to use. Infusions are made by just soaking the leafy material in the liquid we are using, in this case pure water.

We don't want any chemical reaction with our herbal active principles and any substances in the water, so in this case, I recommend using distilled water. You can buy minerals from a health food store to add to the distilled water so it doesn't draw the minerals out of your herbal mixture. The key is keeping everything as natural as possible. You definitely do not want chlorine in the water you are using.

Probably the most important active principle you will be working with for facials is allantoin. It stimulates the growth of new cells. Allantoin is also found in the amniotic fluid surrounding the developing fetus inside a pregnant woman. We want the allantoin to stimulate the growth of your new skin cells. Preparing the herbal mixture is probably the most important part of the entire facial procedure. Please follow these directions exactly.

Comfrey is the most important facial herb. It contains the allantoin and an active form of calcium to stimulate the absorption of the allantoin into the facial skin. It should be picked that day and preferably when the sun is at a peak. The other herbs, plantain leaf, nettle leaf, and lavender flowers are accessory activators of the allantoin.

Use a glass or ceramic pot to boil your water. Do not put the herbs into the pot until it has cooled a bit and is no longer boiling. We are making an infusion and we do not want to boil the leafy herbs. Chop up fresh comfrey leaf, plantain leaf, nettle leaf, and lavender flowers and put them in the warm water in a covered clear glass jar and if possible let the covered jar sit in the sun for an hour or two. The active principles from the herbs should dissolve into the water in the sun. It is ready and should be applied to the face as soon as possible after bringing it in from the sun.

The patient should be laying back and the cotton cloth or pamper type diaper should be soaked in the herbal infusion and applied to the patient's face. Pat it lightly around the entire face so there is maximum contact between the skin and the mixture. You may have to cut an opening in the cloth near the nostrils to allow the patient to breathe. After about 10 minutes add some more of the herbal mixture to the cloth and then again after another ten minutes.

Then remove the herbal pack and let the liquid dry on the skin. After it is dry, do not rinse the face. Use cotton balls to put on a light coating of witch hazel liquid to close the pores. Or make a natural cucumber astringent.

Cucumbers contain natural vegetable hormones which are very beneficial for your skin. Cucumber is also a natural, harmless skin tightener, or astringent. It will do wonders to your wrinkles and lines. Cucumber is used extensively in Sweden and Germany as an active ingredient in commercially manufactured cosmetics

Make 1 cup of fresh cucumber juice from a juice extractor or grate very fine and press through a cloth. Add1/4 of a tsp of honey if you are not vegan. Pour ingredients in an empty bottle, shake well, apply with a cotton ball on your face and neck and refrigerate the leftovers.

Take some drops of Dr. Airola's facial oil and massage it into the face on top of the dried herbal mixture and astringent. Time to relax. Let the blood come to your face and start things working. Just relax for a while.

7. Special facial oil

This is the special formula that Dr. Airola taught us. It should be applied to the face after the facial treatment a few drops at a time massaged into the skin of the face. Hopefully, eventually you will not need to wear any makeup, but if you do, apply a little oil to your skin before you use any makeup.

Some of these items might be a little expensive and if they are just use some cold-pressed sesame oil mixed with a little extra virgin olive oil. All your oils, including the mixtures, must be kept refrigerated. They can go bad soon.

2 tbsp of cold-pressed sesame oil

1 tbsp of extra virgin olive oil

2 tbsp of avocado oil

2 tbsp of almond oil

Pour those oils into a small glass jar that has a cover

Then open the following capsules and drain them into the jar:

2000 IU of natural Vitamin E (5 capsules of 400 IU each)

100,000 USP units of natural Vitamin A (4 capsules of 25,000 units each)

If the vit A has a fishy aroma that bothers you, you can add a few drops of your favorite natural perfume essence, but not cologne.

Shake the mixture well and massage into your face and refrigerate it. The healing oils will revitalize your skin to restore its natural activities. Your complexion will look and feel velvety soft, smooth and lusciously healthy and the physiology of your skin will be restored and rejuvenated.

Acne

Pores become clogged with sebum oil and dirt. Clean it with an oil high in linoleic acid : safflower, black cumin oil, hemp seed oil, pumpkin seed oil, rose hip oil, soybean oil, wheat germ oil and add some of it to your diet.

8. Ingestion

The following section has to do with some nutritional needs for achieving and maintaining a healthful skin appearance. Any nutrient deficiency can eventually result in unattractive skin tone and texture, so eat a well-balanced plant-based diet. Eat a variety of fresh fruits and vegetables every day. Lots of rich color is indicative of the food being rich in nutrients. If you eat well, you normally will not have any conditions and symptoms of deficiencies.

A truly beautiful face exudes health, and that health is due to proper nutrition and a positive outlook on life. Constipation can make the skin appear unhealthy. Actually, any destructive process going on in your body will show up in your face. Any emotional or mental disorder will show also. Part of being beautiful is having wonderful expressions.

Here are some nutrients that especially promote a beautiful appearance.

Sulfur the beauty mineral. Essential for healthy hair, skin, and nails. <u>Natural sources</u>: watercress, onions, radishes, string beans, turnips, celery, horseradish, kale, soybeans.

Silicon fights against the ageing of skin and prevents wrinkles, stops thinning of hair and loss of hair. <u>Natural sources</u>: grapes, beets, onions, horsetail, nettle, alfalfa, strawberries, apples, oats, parsnips, almonds, peanuts, sunflower seeds, kelp, flaxseed

Selenium slows down the aging process in very small doses. May be toxic in large doses. <u>Natural sources</u>: brewer's yeast, sea water, kelp, garlic, mushrooms

Magnesium deficiency of magnesium can cause wrinkles. <u>Natural sources</u>: nuts, soybeans, green leafy vegetables, brown rice, almonds, figs, apples, celery, whole grains, sunflower seeds, alfalfa

Vitamin B15 fights premature aging, regulates fat metabolism. <u>Natural sources</u>: whole grains, seeds, nuts,

Vitamin F promotes healthy skin: <u>Natural sources</u>: soybean oil, flaxseed oil, safflower oil, sunflower seed oil

Pantothenic Acid prevents premature ageing and wrinkles. <u>Natural sources</u>: brewer's yeast, wheat germ, peanuts, molasses, whole grain bread, peas, beans, greens

PABA (vitamin x) essential for healthy skin. <u>Natural sources</u>: brewer's yeast, molasses, wheat germ, whole grains

Vitamin B3 essential for healthy skin. <u>Natural sources</u>: brewer's yeast, wheat germ, brown rice, sunflower seeds, nuts, peanuts, greens

Vitamin A nourishes skin and hair. <u>Natural sources</u>: carrots, greens, squash, cantaloupe, tomatoes, yams

Eat for beauty

Eat some of the following foods to maximize your good health and your beauty will shine through. Millet, buckwheat, sprouts, homemade sauerkraut (uncooked), pickled vegetables, homemade sour pickles, vegetable broth, fruit salads, alfalfa seeds, raw vegetables, raw fruit, mung beans, brewer's yeast, cold-pressed sesame oil (keep refrigerated). Lecithin. Raw potatoes are specifically good for the skin.

Do NOT eat salt, coffee, chocolate, tea, sugar, processed food, synthetic food, refined foods, meat, eggs, cow's milk, or fish

Occasionally do a juice fast

Use the following fresh juices: green vegetable, carrot, beet, celery, spinach, cucumber, black currant, red grape

Herbs for tea: comfrey, burdock, juniper, goldenrod, lavender, slippery elm, strawberry leaves, elecampane.

Try some aloe vera.

Beauty

"A desire to be beautiful is not unwomanly. A woman who is not beautiful cannot properly fill her place. But, mark you, true beauty is not of the face, but of the soul. There is a beauty so deep and lasting that it will shine out of the homeliest face and make it comely. This is the beauty to be first sought and admired. It is a quality of the mind and heart and is manifested in word and deed. A happy heart, a smiling face, loving words and deeds, and a desire to be of service, will make any woman beautiful."

– Mable Hale, Beautiful Girlhood

9. Dr. Cargill's 100% natural cream for severe wrinkles

This takes a little effort to make and you will need some way of blending the materials, either a hand-held blender or a stationary blender. The final product is a cream that can be worked into wrinkles and must be stored in a refrigerator.

Advanced wrinkles can occur on an older face and also on a face that has been exposed to a lot of outdoor weathering. Those wrinkles are deeper than the lighter wrinkles that form on a younger person's face. The deeper wrinkles likely contain some scar tissue which will require special attention and more time to alleviate. The more severe wrinkles must be stretched open and the cream worked into the deepest parts of the wrinkles. It may take a year for severe wrinkles, but isn't it worth it?

Scar tissue is difficult to open so the blood can enter the wrinkle and heal it. Scientists have found that organic zinc molecules can loosen the scar tissue in the wrinkle. So we want to use some material that might contain the organic zinc molecules: onion, brewer's yeast, pumpkin seeds, sunflower seeds, and wheat germ.

In the seeds, the organic zinc is locked up in phytin and must be unlocked by sprouting the seeds. One way to do this is on a damp towel kept reasonably warm for a few days. Maybe it will take a week, but keep the seeds damp and warm and covered so they are in the dark. Use some pumpkin seeds, sunflower seeds, and wheat kernels. You do not want garden seeds because those are treated with chemicals. So get the seeds at a health food store. Hopefully they are alive. If only one type of the seeds sprout, then just use those.

You will need some way of finely chopping the sprouts, preferable in a blender. Add some onion to the mix to be chopped. Maybe one fourth of an onion, 2 TBSP of chopped onion. Use an onion that is not especially strong so it is not uncomfortable on your skin. Cut it from near the center of the onion. Add almost one half a cup of pure water when you are using the blender. Also add 1 TBSP of brewer's yeast. Let it chop and mix thoroughly. When the mixture is liquified, pour off a half cup of the liquid into a container and hopefully strain out most of the solid material. Then discard everything left in the blender and clean it.

Pour the liquid we just made back into the clean blender. Add almost 1/4 cup of pumpkin seed oil, 1/4 cup of sunflower seed oil into the blender. If you do not have both oils then use 1/2 a cup of the oil you do have. Next add a teaspoon of wheat germ oil and a teaspoon of tea tree oil.

When you do the final mix you will need an emulsifier to help form a cream. If you are not vegan add at least 1/2 ounce of pure beeswax and one small egg yolk (preferably a fertile egg) into the blender. If you are vegan, you can purchase a vegetable emulsifier and put in at least 2 TBSP of it. You may have to add more later to thicken the mix into a cream. Mix it well. Don't be in a hurry. Mix it well. Store the cream in a covered jar and refrigerate it.

This cream is specifically for deep wrinkles and pock marks and skin that has been deeply weathered. Put some on your finger and work it deep into the wrinkle and let it stay there. Do it every day. If it is uncomfortable because of the onion juice, then unfortunately you will have to remake the cream. This time leave out the onion or use a milder onion or less onion, but onion is an important ingredient and hopefully you can use it.

Make your skin beautiful again. Your well-being is worth it. When you look better, you will feel better. Be patient. Natural healing takes time.